Stop Codependency

How to End the Vicious Cycle of Codependent Relationships, Stop Manipulative Behavior in Its Tracks, and Learn to Love Yourself and Others in a Real Healthy Relationship

Antony Felix

Your Free Gift

As a way of thanking you for the purchase, I'd like to offer you a complimentary gift:

- **5 Pillar Life Transformation Checklist:** This short book is about life transformation, presented in bit size pieces for easy implementation. I believe that without such a checklist, you are likely to have a hard time implementing anything in this book and any other thing you set out to do religiously and sticking to it for the long haul. It doesn't matter whether your goals relate to weight loss, relationships, personal finance, investing, personal development, improving communication in your family, your overall health, finances, improving your sex life, resolving issues in your relationship, fighting PMS successfully, investing, running a successful business, traveling etc. With a checklist like this one, you can bet that anything you do will seem a lot easier to implement until the end. Therefore, even if you don't continue reading this book, at least read the one thing that will help you in every other aspect of your life. Grab your copy now by clicking/tapping here or simply enter http://bit.ly/2fantonfreebie into your browser. Your life will never be the same again (if you implement what's in this book), I promise.

PS: I'd like your feedback. If you are happy with this book, please leave a review on Amazon.

Introduction

This book has actionable information on how to end the vicious cycle of codependent relationships, stop manipulative behavior in its tracks and learn to love yourself and others in a real healthy relationship.

Do you live with someone suffering a bad addiction or some sort of irresponsibility behavior that they seem can't help overcome? Do you, on the other hand, out of something you can't understand, maybe love - so you think (or pity), feel so attached to this person and therefore obliged to take up his problems as yours?

Do you do this just to make him or her feel good about you and win their approval? Do you go to an extent of contemplating bearing the consequences of their wrong deeds? Worse still, have they started reciprocating your 'kind' deeds towards them by being manipulative instead? The situation is complex, but does it sound synonymous with you or someone you know?

Well, those are just but a few red alerts of a deep-seated relationship called codependency. By helping you understand this problem, this book puts you first on a self-examination path.

It then gives you a manual to use to overcome this unhealthy relationship cycle. It guides you into self-appreciation, freedom from this slavery and puts you along the path of self-love, as the true basis of loving and helping others effectively.

Table of Contents

Stop Codependency

Chapter 1: What is Codependency?

What comes to mind when you read the word 'codependency'?

The answer is a relationship thriving on mutual benefits.

Well, interestingly, nothing could be so wrong than that answer because, there're actually no tangible positive results in this relationship. On the contrary, it's only detrimental to both parties.

The motive behind this relationship is where the problem lies.

Codependency is described as a relationship where one person continues sacrificing his or her needs and times to meet someone else's needs of coping with the challenges of his or her (often irresponsible) way of life.

Since the root cause of the problem of the person being helped is not met, the problem persists, availing the need for more help and the partner goes on helping.

In other terms, it involves creating an 'enabling relationship' where both partners help each other to continue doing what they do to sustain a codependency relationship.

Take an example with an addict shoplifter...

Apparently, a certain bloke cannot help shoplifting occasionally. In several occasions, he has even been made to do odd things from cleaning a whole store to paying huge fines as punishment but he always slides back to the vice.

You, on the other hand, as the partner, has become the understanding one, the enabler; offering him a helping hand whenever faced with a punishment. You even helped pay fines. Apparently, you enjoy helping this addict but in the process of sympathizing with him, you're not helping to tame the vice.

You're enabling him to continue. His addiction depends on your support and your support depends on his addiction – codependency.

What Motivates You To Help?

Although your intentions of actually helping someone cope with challenging life seems good, it's only about decade ago that it was discovered they're not actually driven by the need to help, but by the need to address your very own insecurities, your self-worth, your low self-esteem.

In a nutshell, it's about trying to meet the needs of someone else so that you can feel needed and valued.

By enabling others cope with their problems, you're actually looking to win their approval and that of the public too. You believe that by working so hard to alleviate the suffering of someone whom the society seems helpless about, you win the hearts of many.

That gives you an approval rating and a sense of self-worth. That's exactly what drives you into codependency relationship to become an enabler; a benefactor. However, the day this relationship starts weighing on you and brings no positive change to your partner, it starts becoming a toxic one and repercussions become evident.

So what are the consequences? Let's discuss that.

Consequences of Codependency

Although your aim in offering a helping hand is to minimize the bad effects of addiction and gain some marks for yourself - good for self-esteem - it always does not help things in that direction. Your actions unfortunately are actually fostering even more addiction.

When the partner sees that help is always forthcoming whenever needed, he continues in his old style of doing things like an addict to ensure more and more help and care is coming.

For example, when you act the codependent and easily give in to the whims of a drug addict child to stay at home and not help with chores, and be manipulated by the child's many excuses including threats of self-harm when you force them do what they don't want, that can only serve to sink the child deeper into addiction.

Your efforts of helping them out of the situation therefore become meaningless. This takes a toll on your already fragile self-esteem.

The addict partner on the other hand takes your deliberate repeated rescue efforts as a right for him. He therefore continues expecting them from you while continuing in their self-destructive behavior of self-indulgence into their specific addiction.

More so, they may want to manipulate you into the direction you should take to help them further. Theirs become an unspoken demand for the good treatment. But these are only the general consequences to expect. There could be even some more effects and they include:

1: Mental health issues – When your efforts are rejected each time you try to help an addict, you become frustrated. The frustration of not being able to convince your abuser or the person you are codependent on to agree to pay heed to your advice and improve on his behavior is likely to add to your routine stress. This stress builds up and turns into chronic stress, which sabotages your mental wellbeing.

Anxiety is another commonly experienced offshoot in a codependent relationship. Being the victim of codependency, it is likely that the abuser takes out the brunt of his/ her negativity on you. Every time you sense something may upset him/ her, trigger his/ her addiction or set off his/ her volatile behavior, you are likely to become scared. This state, if not managed, too can result in panic attacks, which can aggravate your anxiousness and make you succumb to an anxiety disorder.

Depression is another consequence of being in a codependent relationship. When you are isolated by your abuser or are constantly emotionally, physically or sexually abused him/her or are manipulated to the extent that you feel insane yourself, you are likely to feel withdrawn and dejected which can turn into depression. Moreover, you can also experience self-harming thoughts including suicidal thoughts primarily because you feel there is no end to your misery and that it may only end with you departing the world.

All these issues only lower your already strained self-esteem. Your opinion and value of yourself keeps depleting with each passing day and insecurity soon takes over you.

Many people suffering in codependent relationships feel they are incompetent and do not deserve to be happy because of the constant manipulation and ill treatment suffered at the hands of their abuser.

2. Physical health problems- The stress, anxiety, depression and other mental health problems you experience can quickly lead to other health concerns namely hypertension (high blood pressure), ulcers, headaches and possibly heart problems. Stress is one of the biggest contributors of high blood pressure, diabetes and cardiovascular disorders.

Moreover, the stress and anxiety you experience can also pave way for eating disorders. You may start stuffing food on top of your stress to shove it deep inside you so you do not feel it; or you may start starving yourself for long periods because the chronic stress, anxiety and depression you experience suppress your hunger.

If you suffer from chronic stress, which goes unaddressed for a long time period, your likelihood of developing any one or more of these health conditions increases too and this greatly lowers the quality of your life.

3. Addiction to alcohol and drugs – Most people run away from frustrations by drowning themselves alcohol and drugs. When you have to deal with codependency frustrations, you might easily slip into substance and alcohol abuse and easily become addicted. This compounds the problem of codependency even further making it even more difficult for you to save yourself from the abuse and live a happy life.

4. Relationship problems – Notice that the aim of you getting involved in a codependency relationship in the first place is to establish a good strong relationship with the partner and people around you – to earn your place in society as a helper and a problem solver. But then here you're and your efforts bear no fruits. You will soon start viewing yourself a looser and people around you won't give you much credit for your effort and if any, it will only be pity and empathy for you. That already creates a relationship tension, as people will start viewing you differently. Not only that, but when you are constantly controlled, abused and negatively influenced by someone you share a codependent relationship, your behavior is likely to become strange, withdrawn and negative with others as well. You may not be as laid back or fun as you were before with your friends. You may start acting out more with your kids venting out your frustration on them. You may lose your calm on the pettiest of issues with everyone around you. Your professional relationships may get the brunt of it too with you not socializing much with people, reaching out to your networks on time and not responding efficiently to your boss's orders and arguing with him/ her when you are not supposed to. All of this only negatively affects your relationships adding more to your misery.

5. Picking Up on Negative Behaviors and Addictions- This is a commonly suffered and a possible outcome of being in a codependent relationship. When you live with a drug addict or someone who emotionally, sexually or physically abuses you, or a narcissist, or with someone who controls you negatively through different means, it is likely that you may pick up on any of his/ her bad behaviors sooner or later. If that person is a liar, maybe you develop that character trait with time as well; or if he/ she is into drug abuse, you may turn into a junkie as well. There is always the risk of following the footsteps of your abuser because you spend a great deal of time with him/ her on a daily basis.

6. Poor Productivity and Performance in Different Aspects of Life - When you are constantly subjected to manipulating, maltreatment and abuse in a number of forms, it takes a toll on your emotional wellbeing and even physical health. Naturally, when you do not feel fit mentally and physically, you are not able to properly focus on any of your tasks and your performance is likely to become poorer with time. This gradually decreases your productivity and you stop doing well in different areas of your life, primarily your career.

Is the Codependency Condition Permanent?

Well, for starters, the good news is that there is no evidence linking codependency to any disease.

However, often, health care and mental wellbeing experts and psychologists refer to codependency as a disease because alcoholism or drug addiction is often involved in it.

Moreover, since codependency is progressive, experiencing it is similar to suffering from a disease. As those around us get sicker, we start reacting with heightened intensity. What may have begun as a small concern is likely to set off depression, isolation, physical illness, emotional problems or worst case scenario- suicidal fantasies.

One problem leads to another and before you realize it, the situation becomes seriously aggravated. While codependency is not an actual illness, it does have the power to make you feel extremely sick.

However, in reality, the condition is simply a grossly immoral cycle brought about by an acquired behavior and brain conditioning. Being a form of entanglement, an emotional slavery of sort, the condition is reversible and therefore not permanent. You only need to self-evaluate and denounce the vice out of you in the strongest terms that we are soon going to learn in the next chapter.

Unfortunately, although it can be done, turning a codependency relationship around in a simple perfunctory DIY may be difficult. A meticulous DIY therapy process is the ideal option for an entire change from codependency.

We'll see exactly how you can actively break the addiction in our next chapter covering codependency recovery.

Who Is Likely To Be In A Codependent Relationship?

Individuals who find themselves surviving a codependency relationship are mostly those brought up a in a dysfunctional family.

Such is a family where conflict, child abuse, child neglect and misdemeanors by parents become so rampant to a point that these vices acquired a normal view and got acquiesced especially by the children. Children may develop some notions that they are the reason their parents are so abusive to them. They therefore feel they must do something about it and the only thing is to serve the needs of their abusive (maybe alcoholics) parents to the letter so that they win acceptance and approval from them and possibly end the bad treatment.

The children grow up with a sense of a compulsive duty to subvert their own needs and protect and serve the needs of their parents or other siblings. This is also done in the context that the problems of their families are never to be aired away to public attention. Failure to do so makes the 'caretaker' child feel like a failure and worthless and that affects his or her esteem and self-worth a lot. In other words, children depend on their parents' undoing to get an opportunity to build their self-worth.

That is how codependents are born.

Later in life, when such children encounter anyone else in need of their attention, they find it in them that unless they take upon themselves and help out, they will continue feeling guilty and suffer neglect from society.

Are you such kind of person? Perhaps you may want to self-test to determine whether you suffer from codependency. Let's discuss more about this.

Chapter 2: Codependency Tests: Are You Codependent?

So far, you have learnt what the making behind a codependent is. You're determined this must not continue but first, you badly want to know whether you or a friend you suspect could actually be in a codependent relationship. This you will easily know by picking out specific signs and symptoms.

You could also conduct a codependency test online where popular websites such as <u>Wining-Teams</u> or <u>Souls Shepherding</u> among others offer quick quizzes to test your codependency status.

<u>http://www.winning-teams.com/codependent_test.html</u>

<u>http://www.soulshepherding.org/2005/07/codependency-test/</u>

The questionnaire focuses on exploring the signs and symptoms of this relationship with you in view. It's only by self-examining through such a checklist that you will be able to know where you stand in this kind of relationship.

After that, it will be easier to cut yourself off from the cycle.

As you conduct the tests, keep in mind that probable signs and symptoms that you are codependent will often include:

1. **Taking responsibility of others' misbehaviors and misdeeds** – This is the top behavior for codependents and you should reject it. It could be a brother and because he is always drunk and can't help it to stop, he occasionally goes on rampage in the market destroying traders' wares and insulting the masses. Before he's lynched, you the enabler, quickly jump in and strongly defend and rescue him and literary offer to take the responsibility. That could be the height of codependency relationship.

2. **People pleasing** leading to a struggle in attending to your own needs – due to a deep-seated urge to please, you find yourself neglecting or compromising your own needs and happiness to attend to other people's first. You do those for fear of rejection because if you can stand up to face your partner and tell them the truth, they will reject you.

   The end result is that you end up suffering because it finally gets too late to attend to your own problems.

3. **Feeling inadequate in your own life outside a specific someone** – Due to the attachment that exists between codependents, you may feel at odds if your partner is away from you and for long. You may want to always keep in touch, on phone or so and you always feel inadequate in their absence – something more of an obsession than love.

4. **Being overprotective of your codependent** – You find yourself protecting an irresponsible person. After that, you rush to help them deal with the problem because you know there isn't a way they are able to handle the matter on their own. Reject this tendency.

5. **You continue staying with someone** despite his or her unhealthy behavior – because you want to validate some help for someone, you cannot stay away from him or her. People wonder how you cope but to you, it's a duty you must accomplish because apparently, you believe you will earn people's approval from that noble duty.

6. **Offering advice, even unsolicited one**, to someone so regularly – because as a helper in a codependent relationship, you're always keen to the problems of an addict; you quickly jump in to opportunity to offer helpful advice now and then.

7. **Feeling angry and unappreciated** when people don't seem to recognize your efforts – whenever you help someone out of a self-afflicted problem, you tend to wait for applause. If then even the slightest recognition is not forthcoming, you feel emotionally harmed, sad and angry.

8. **Want to feel you're in control** – One trait with codependents is that you gauge how you influence everyone's behavior around you. You always want to feel in control of people's behavior around you by subtly devising ways of making people feel guilty, and shame for

not tending to an addict. That is the manipulative tactic that always works for you to ensure you are in control.

9. **Never really open up to people about your true self** – If you badly fear that people might disapprove your suggestions or actions, you never really share or open up to people about yourself well. You dread being exposed because apparently how you present yourself outwardly as a sincere helper is not exactly who you are but someone only helping others to gain approval.

To help you understand how 'addictive' codependency can get, let's take a look at the cycle of codependence in a relationship.

The Vicious Cycle Of A Codependence Relationship

This cycle of needing to seek outside confirmation from your partner that you are good enough certainly starts somewhere. If you could master the cycle and the triggers, things can get pretty easy for you. For starters, understand that it is a process that occurs in mind.

Let's consider a relationship where, for the fear of being left by your partner, you feel compelled to be personally responsible for their general wellbeing.

The cycle unfolds as follows:

1. Everything seems okay in your relationship.

2. The okay state of affairs gets a bit boring and a sense of insecurity creeps in your mind. It says *'you are not doing pretty enough for your partner in terms of ensuring his or her happiness, wants, feelings or general wellbeing'*.

3. You then act accordingly and endeavor to inculcate into your partner what you think will make them appreciate you.

4. Partner responds in a dramatic, rather vigorously, way and a fight may ensue putting both of you in a hormone rage. During the fight, there are fears of abandonment contempt and shame in you.

5. While this dramatic response lasts, you together realize you cannot continue like that and hence come into a truce of sort. Things apparently get back to 'okay' status again. But remember nothing has yet been resolved in terms of the original fears you had of insecurity. If anything, they have been worsened.

6. Soon, the temporary relief fades away and in a precedent turn of events, you as the insecure partner in the relationship repeats step one and the cycle continues.

Codependency also creates a hormonal imbalance in your body, which disrupts the normal flow of mood improving hormones such as dopamine and serotonin and that of stress triggering hormones adrenaline and cortisol.

This hormonal imbalance too makes you behave strangely. You may feel more depressed, which increases your dependency for approval on your manipulator, which makes you stick to the relationship longer.

Additionally, the highs and lows of a codependent relationship make you immune to it and you become accustomed to receiving good and bad treatment from your manipulator. When you build a habit of it, you want the same treatment over and over from that person when you do not receive it, which increases your dependency on your abuser.

As it's apparent from the cycle above, the clingier you become to a partner, the easier it is for them to counter attack from the point of pride. Stop being jealous, obsessed and controlling to a partner; embrace self-sufficiency and trust and stop the 'needy' tag. It could be easier than done though.

In the next chapter, you will learn the vital steps you should take towards full recovery.

Chapter 3: How To Break The Chains Of Codependency

The top reason why you may be suffering alone in a relationship as someone with a lost identity is ignorance about how to break the vicious cycle of unhealthy relationship - codependence. You do not want to confront the problem for the anxiety, stress and fear of being left alone if you anger your partner.

You also could be of the opinion that you are responsible for your partner's happiness and if you leave the relationship, something unforeseen may befall them. However, you can step outside of this uncomfortable 'comfort' zone, examine your relationship pattern and discover that whatever has been ailing your relationship has a cure and the cure is within you.

A DIY Recovery Process From Codependency Relationship

The journey to full recovery from problems that started from childhood days can be long but it certainly starts somewhere.

For a quick healing from this vicious and unhealthy cycle of codependency in a relationship, the overall lesson is learning how to make your needs priority; avoiding the 'insecurity' malady.

Below is a DIY guide that will help you overcome the insecurities and fears that trigger the codependency relationship cycle.

1: Learn to accept you've a problem

In an ideal relationship setting, each partner must address his/her own needs like health and happiness in order to be able to serve the other partner effectively. If you self-neglect for the sake of others' wellbeing, then there is a problem. Acknowledging that you've a problem will set the need in you to recover.

However, often times, as a codependent, you do not realize you have a problem, a problem of disregarding your emotions and feelings and putting others' ahead of yours. Therefore, accepting that you have been living on self-denial is not easy. You can, however, learn to accept that you have a problem in the following two ways.

✓ **Interrogate your true emotions** – Ask yourself whether you really act to please others with an exclusion of your own self or you do so to please both. You will realize the more times you support your partner, the more you get disappointed with results and the more people don't seem to appreciate you. Whenever you feel upset, frustrated, depressed, angry, anxious, jealous, happy, excited or any other emotion in reference to your manipulator, question your emotions and their authenticity over and over again. For instance, if you feel happy when your abusive partner praises you, ask yourself if you actually feel happy or is it accompanied by underlying guilt because you know you are only tricking yourself into feeling happy and do not really feel good about being with that person? Similarly, if you feel fury built inside you every time your abuser gaslights you, controls you or isolates you, dig deeper into the rage and figure out the message it is trying to convey to you. It is likely it intends to communicate to you the misery you are engulfed in and so wish to come out of.

✓ **List some good deeds you have done to yourself in the recent past** – if none, and most likely it is none for enablers in codependent relationships; realize then you have a problem catering to yourself.

✓ **Focus on your feelings**- dig deeper into your feelings to better understanding how you really feel about yourself and the life you are living currently. Ask yourself questions like: Am I truly happy living this life? Is this the reality I wanted for myself? Is this the happiness I dreamt of? How does being with that person really make me feel? How do I feel about my life? Is there something about my life that I would like to change? Why do not I feel alive from within? Dig deeper into these questions and reflect on their answers by writing down your feelings or even recording them. The deeper you delve into them, the more you realize how wretched you feel and how that dejection is brought about by the controlling person you are sharing a close relationship with.

✓ **Accept your condition out aloud and write it down**- when you are sure you are living in a codependent relationship, it is important to acknowledge it out aloud and even better, in writing. Just like a doctor's diagnosis confirms your health issue or disease and you instantly become more concerned about your health, a written declaration of being in a codependent relationship makes you more conscious of the problem at hand and makes you actively work towards resolving the issue. Now you need to say out aloud that you are in a codependent relationship and wish to escape the pain. You could phrase the statement in any way you like such as '*I am living in a codependent relationship with (name of relationship) and I wish to live a healthier, happier life by breaking this vicious cycle of codependency.*' Speak this statement out aloud at least 10 times very clearly, slowly, loudly and confidently so it rings in your ears and you actually hear yourself say and feel it. This makes you consciously accept the problem and become more determined to work on it.

✓ **Think of how happy life can become**- After acknowledging your problem, give yourself more reason to actively work on breaking the vicious codependency cycle by thinking of how beautiful and meaningful life can actually become if you break free of the abuse you suffer from every single day of your life. Ponder on how free and calm you will feel when there is nobody to manipulate you and make you act like their puppet. Think of how you will have the option of doing everything you ever wanted to do because now there is nobody you have to unwillingly look after or take orders from. Think of how you won't have to suffer from physical, sexual and psychological abuse at the hands of your abuser every other day because you have eliminated that toxicity from your life. Ponder on how self-assured and secure you will feel because you will actually get a chance to focus on your own needs and self-care, something you have deprived yourself of for a very long time. Focus on how for a change you will get to be the actual boss of your life instead of a slave who is living his/ her life while obeying the commands of someone else. Think of how you won't be crying every other hour, feeling pain stab your heart every day and being isolated from all the happiness you can actually enjoy. Think of how you will feel calmer, confident, relaxed, poised, happy, peaceful and motivated from within and how all of that will help you follow your dreams, take care of yourself, spend quality time with positive people, focus on your wellbeing and live life on your terms. Focus on how you will actually reclaim your life and become empowered from within once you bid adieu to your abuser. This will certainly motivate you to end that codependent relationship and become free. To liberate yourself from the pain, do write down all the compelling reasons that encourage you to pull the plug and move on with your life. Having a goal and not accompany it with compelling reasons is similar to not having a real goal at all. Make sure yours is a meaningful, complete goal by pegging compelling reasons to it. These motivate you to stick to the goal when your willpower depletes and you feel like calling it quits. In such times, it is these reasons and a written account of them that convinces you to get back on the saddle and race one more time because you have got to make it to the finish line.

Be honest to yourself and to whoever matters to you about your true emotions and feelings. You now need to go through this account over and over again, at least once daily to remind yourself of the new mission you have embarked on to save yourself from the harms of the codependent relationship you have been living in for years.

2: Recognize and detach yourself from the obsessions

Your next task is to distance yourself from that person and let go of the need to constantly feel obsessed about him/ her and take care of all his/ her needs. This doesn't mean you are avoiding responsibility; it just means you have an unhealthy obsession that you must sacrifice and drop for your own good.

But how will you know you're obsessed to something?

✓ If most of your time is spent thinking about the thing or person, it is likely you are obsessed about him/ her. Also, pay attention to what you think about when thinking about him/ her. Do you genuinely miss him/ her or are you more concerned about how he/ she will function without you and how infuriated he/ she may become when he/ she does not find you around or does not get any of his needs fulfilled with you not being around to take care of him/ her? If it is the latter and you feel compelled to be around him/ her, it is likely you are obsessed about him/ her and that comes from all the manipulation you have been exposed to.

✓ If you sacrifice your needs to attend to someone or something else, and feel miserable about it, it is clear you are being controlled by that person which has now made you obsessive about him/ her. Making compromises and letting go of your demands some times, even your important needs to please the other person or make him/ her feel special is alright in any important and close relationship if that happens occasionally. However, this becomes abnormal if it is done on a daily basis and if you are somehow forced or made to feel that you must sacrifice your wellbeing, needs and self to prioritize the other person and make him/ her feel important. That is not okay and is a HUGE sign of a controlling relationship.

✓ If you can go an extra mile and suffer consequences of partners undoing without much complaining, this too shows you are obsessed about the other person. While you may not complain explicitly, you do not feel good about suffering from within and cringe every time you have to compromise your wellbeing for that person who does not even care how you feel and has no empathy towards you.

✓ If you are constantly reminding yourself of how that controlling person you are living with loves you, cares about you and genuinely wishes to be with you only to make yourself feel better while you know how the reality and evidences do not support this, you are obsessed about him/ her because of the manipulation you have suffered from over a long time. Codependency can turn you into an addict of that person, which makes you feel that the other person is your god and that he/ she cares the most about you. This is how you trick yourself into continuing living with him/ her every time you decide to escape the trauma you are exposed to. This happens due to the constant manipulation you have been subjected to which makes you numb to the pain and makes you feel that this is how you are supposed to live.

You need to observe your behavior for these signs over a period of 5 to 10 days and if you spot any of these, it is likely you are constantly obsessive over that person who does not even care much about it or is maybe under the influence of drugs or some other addiction, which keeps him/ her from being compassionate around you or anybody else.

You now need to step out of this cycle of constantly worrying about that person and start working on yourself. It means you letting your partner suffer the consequences of his or her irresponsibility alone until they learn the hard way if that is what it will take. It may mean saying no where you could readily say yes when your heart feels it's a no. Sometimes it can be easy said than done but with determination, you can do it.

Here are a few good places to slowly detach yourself from that person.

• Make a list of all your needs and prioritize them in the order of their importance starting from most important and moving to least important.

• You then need to slowly focus on one need at a time and constantly remind yourself of the importance of your own self-care. Think of all the times when you need support from your partner or the person you are constantly obsessing over, but he/ she never comes to your aid. Think of all the times you were in pain because of him/ her, but he/ she completely failed to recognize that. When there is nobody to really understand your pain, misery and agony, why do you feel obliged to become intensely

34

concerned about them. Like Buddha once said, '*You of all the people deserve your love and attention the most*', so you need to understand that, accept that and acknowledge it by prioritizing your self-care first. So if you have not rested properly in a long time, do so and take as many naps as you feel like. If that is not possible in your own house because of that controlling person, crash at a friend's place for a night or two or book a hotel room or Air BnB for a couple of hours and just relax.

- Start becoming firm with that controlling person and every time he/ she gives you an instruction which is appalling for you, say no. Be firm, but polite when you do so and clearly communicate your feelings to him/ her about that response. Let him/ her know how that upsets you and that you are no longer going to be his/ her punching bag. In case he/ she is abusive, tell him/ her you have contacted the authorities and will report his/ her behavior instantly. If your manipulator is a drug addict or is incapable of defending himself/ herself, he/ she is likely to budge down on this threat. If he/ she is more influential, it is best not to initiate this argument with him/ her unless you have actually made up your mind to leave him/ her and have contacted the authorities.

- Surround yourself with positive, caring and influential people who genuinely love you and care about you. There is likely to be at least one such person in your life, probably someone who is aware of your condition for a long time and has been warning you about it for quite some time. Reach out to him/ her and talk to him/ her in depth about your feelings, how you wish to escape the trauma and how you would like for him/ her to support you. If he/ she genuinely cares about you, he/ she will instantly agree to help you out.

- Ask him/ her to keep reminding you of how you need to focus on your own wellbeing by keeping a check on your feelings and taking a daily report from you of how you looked after yourself. This may feel exhausting to you at first because you do not have a habit of talking about yourself, but when every day or every other day, you talk about how you paid attention to your needs with someone and share your feelings with them, you will start enjoying this attention and will become more motivated to look after yourself.

- With that person's support, you now need to craft a plan to escape the abuse and manipulation you underwent. Think of the time for which you will test your controlling partner or the manipulative person you share any other close relationship with. If you are living with an addict, maybe getting him/ her into a rehabilitation center will help. If he/ she is not into substance abuse, but suffers from a psychological problem that he/ she does not admit to, you need to observe his/ her behavior for some time and if it does not improve, you need to leave him/ her. To make sure you are able to reach that point, you first need to gather all your important documents such as your passport, ID card, medical certificates, insurance documents and any other important documents that may be in that person's custody when he/ she is way. Get copies of those documents and give the originals to your supportive friend. Get a spare phone and sim card for the time when you leave your controller and hand it to your friend.

3: Stop enabling and start supporting out

In the context of codependency, enabling encourages the addiction to continue, while supporting out ensures that the partner is able to come out of the addiction. The problem is that you have been an enabler and not a supporter, which is why the situation has worsened to this extent where you feel completely blocked and controlled by the other person and have nowhere to go. Help your partner overcome their problem if its pride, insecurity addition or anything. Do not allow the status quo to continue by making the circumstances conducive.

Try out the following tricks for supporting your partner out of the addiction.

✓ Stop sympathizing with your partner on his actions; focus more on yourself and detach from helping your partner with his or her problem. Let them bear the consequences of their actions alone. This may spell to your partner to 'be responsible of your own actions, you are alone' and soon will start developing a sense of responsibility. If he/ she does not stop taking drugs and finds a way to sneak them into your house, be firm with him/ her and throw the drugs out and even that person for some time if you have to, even if it is your kid. It is going to be hard, but you have to be firm and let him/ her know you are not going to buy their tricks anymore. If he/ she asks you for money, do not lend them any. If your refusal makes him/ her act abusively or resort to assaulting you, call the police immediately. That ought to give him/ her a clear message how you are not going to take any abuse from him/ her now and are determined to live better and not encourage their negative demeanor anymore.

✓ Do not abandon your partner entirely; addicts are vulnerable and know that they could be a nuisance to society. If you abandon them, they may confirm they are actually a problem to people and will most likely delve even more into their addiction, substance abuse, or gambling addiction, for example. You just need to be firm with him/ her and communicate your concerns with him/ her in a strict tone. You must not also give in to their whims and wishes, but at this stage, do not leave him/ her instantly. It is best to stick around for a little longer, observe his/ her behavior and make one last attempt to help him/ her improve. That said, if he/ she becomes severely abusive and assaults you, you would have to abandon him/ her.

✓ Stop forcing/pushing treatment ideas to an addict; understand that any addict is also not so happy about themselves being addicted. They know they could be a nuisance to people and because apparently they can help it, they may want to counter any attacks directed at them with fierce defense for themselves. Like a psychiatrist case, the approach to introducing any treatment idea to an addict partner should be gradual and subtle. Be friendly in the approach. Talk to him/ her about the importance of living a clean, safe and happy life and how overcoming their addiction will help them actualize that goal. Remind him/ her of how his/ her life is a gift, one that needs to be taken care of and how he/ she is missing out on a lot by letting their addiction wash them over. With that, introduce him/ her to the concept of incremental goals, which refers to setting small goals for every day or week of the recovery plan instead of trying to quit instantly and taking that goal as one, huge chunk. For instance, if your child, partner or sibling is addicted to booze, decide a certain span of time both of you think will be enough for him/ her to give up on the addiction. Usually, 6 to 12 months are enough, but pick a duration keeping in mind that person's personality, behavior and the pace at which he/ she works. Next, set a small goal for every week of the 3 or 6 or 9 months recovery plan. For instance, if your partner drinks about 10 bottles of alcohol every day, encourage him to drink 8 a day for 2 weeks and then move to 6 bottles a day in the third week and then 5 bottles in the fourth week and then 3 bottles a day in the fifth week and then 1 bottle a week in the sixth week. From the seventh week onwards, encourage him/ her to shift to glasses instead of bottles a day. As you slowly encourage him/ her to reduce his/ her consumption of alcohol, introduce more coping strategies that help him/ her distract from his/ her temptation and improve his/ her discipline, mental health and physical fitness such as meditation, yoga, exercise, engaging in a sport, listening to good music, reading good books on self-development and recovery, building healthy habits etc. You need to very slowly and gradually make him/ her move towards recovery instead of compelling him/ her to become disciplined at once because the latter is actually impossible.

Understand that no addict will admit they are addicted. Just approach the topic in the line of *'it is important you stop early before it gets too late, to a point of addiction'* even though they are already addicted. Such an approach may allow some sense of listening in them.

4: Explore your childhood experiences

Getting to the bottom of a problem is crucial because that helps you understand your issue better and also the point from where it stems from. If you don't know that you are allergic to peanuts, you may continue to eat them and aggravate your allergies. It is only when you identify the root cause that you steer clear of it and are able to take better care of yourself accordingly. Similarly, to put an end to the vicious codependency cycle you have borne, you now need to dig deeper into cause and figure out from where the problem actually started out. It gives you a reference point and debunks the notion of a mystery problem.

What you went through during your formative years could be the trigger of all the insecurities in you. Although it is not easy to admit that you actually had a disturbing upbringing that is affecting you today, accepting this reality helps you come to terms with the experiences you had then and relate them to your current problems and devise a more effective solution.

But how exactly will you explore your childhood experiences then relate them to your current life? Here are some tips to do that appropriately.

✓ *Revisit what you can remember about your childhood experiences* – some pointers of a kid growing up in a codependent family in caretaker roles, drunk parents, absent parents, very strict and punishing parents.

    o Caretaker roles – If you can recall eras in your childhood where you were left the custody of your siblings while you were a little child yourself and did not have parents or any guardian around to take care of you and those you were given the responsibility of, that could be an indicator of why today you still carry on the roles of a caretaker. You most probably did this to please parents and your siblings of course and you did it so diligently that you even sacrificed your own needs. Maybe you enjoyed the attention and appreciation you received a couple of times when you took care of the little babies in your house whether they were your biological siblings or step ones or cousins who were staying at your house. That attention may have made you feel like an adult, which you enjoyed and wanted to experience time and again, which made you soon nurture the habit of looking after them and taking care of them. However, you did not realize at that point that you were still too young to take up that responsibility because that came with a lot of obligations, which you were not ready to bear.

o Drunken, absent parents – If you were brought up in a family where the duty of keeping things in order at home was yours, because your parents were always away or were wasted majority of the time or just did not care enough to look after you and your siblings, you could have developed the insecurity and pleasing tendencies. While you wanted to please your absent parents with obedience, you wanted them to change but instead they carried on with their absenteeism. You may have also realized how nonchalant they were about you and your siblings, and since someone had to take care of them, you stepped up to bear that responsibility selflessly.

o The environment you were exposed to- If you were exposed to an environment that contained any strong, influencing factors that shaped your personality in a certain manner, that too could be a contributor towards your care giving behavior and your tendency to be easily manipulated. Maybe you grew up seeing your mother look after your abusive father with utmost care, devotion and selflessness to the point that she suffered from it, but never openly spoke about it making you believe that it is the way wives are supposed to behave. Or maybe you read some books or watched movies on dark romance wherein a protagonist is in love with a manipulative person, but is too scared to lose him/ her so suffers all the abuse in silence. This may make you nurture distorted beliefs about love, which have now influenced your behavior, decisions and life greatly. Or maybe you lived in a strongly patriarchal society where you were taught from a young age on how women must make sacrifices in relationships; or maybe you grew up seeing how parents always sacrificed their wellbeing for their kids and supported their kids even if they turned out to be felons or addicts. Such factors and environment is quite likely to make you nurture distorted and unhealthy beliefs, which influence your mindset making you bear with a codependent relationship for quite a long while.

✓ *Ask around about how you were brought up* – If you cannot recall, ask around from other family members. Make notes of every tiny bit of information you receive and try to connect all the puzzle pieces together to make better sense of the entire situation. The more you dig into your childhood, the more knowledge you will attain on how you were brought up and what really influenced your behavior and turn you into a people pleaser and a caregiver who is now suffering from an abusive relationship.

If you surely can relate your current life to your upbringing, you will come to terms with your experiences.

5: Learn to self-communicate

This involves becoming aware of your own feelings, needs and thoughts and then communicating them to your partner and also acknowledging your needs and thoughts yourself and working towards them.

But how exactly do you become self-aware? There are a number of ways to that have been documented and you can try a few.

✓ Mindfulness meditation – because as a codependent, you have almost completely lost contact with your inner self, mindfulness helps you reconnect with your inner self. You become aware of your own thoughts and emotions and you gain some control over them. Mindfulness mediation doesn't take hard practice and is quite an easy practice that you can conveniently perform on your own and then build a habit of it to reap its benefits in your everyday life. But first, it is important to learn what mindfulness meditation actually is and does for you. Mindfulness refers to being in the moment peacefully and nonjudgmentally and accepting each moment as it comes. So whatever you experience within a certain moment, you acknowledge and accept it without bashing it or yourself for experiencing it and then look for ways to appropriately respond to any issues experienced within that time. For instance, if you feel angry, you do not label your anger as a negative emotion, neither do you react to it, but you allow it to soothe on its own while embracing it and exploring it deeper so you figure out what exactly caused it. When you realize it, it is because you have not achieved anything in life because you are busy being manipulated by someone and taking care of them while all your friends are living the life of your dreams, you accept the issue and then find ways to resolve it effectively instead of feeling frustrated by it. The frustration that comes along is accepted as a natural response, but you do not let it get to your head. Neither do you keep rehashing the past and blame yourself for making wrong decisions some years back, but you live in the moment, understand your feelings and seek better ways to best handle them. Mindfulness is actually a state of mind that allows you to live in the present happily while letting go of your past worries and future concerns. This is what makes you aware of how you truly feel instead of letting other emotions such as guilt, fear and shame override them. You need to inculcate a state of mindfulness to become conscious of yourself, your feelings and your behavior to liberate yourself from a traumatic life. Mindfulness is what will help you become aware of your caregiving behaviors every time you willingly agree to succumb to your manipulator's influence so you can put a stop to it on time. One of the best tools to inculcate mindfulness is meditation. It is a practice that can be performed in a number of ways and is carried out with the aim of promoting mindfulness, awareness, peacefulness and complete bliss. It regulates the different brainwaves your brain functions in and improves your ability to think, focus and concentrate on things. Moreover, as it improves the functioning of your brain, your brain is then able to regulate the many other important processes and functions taking place in your body, which improves your overall physical and mental health. Mindfulness based meditation is the best way to inculcate a state of mindfulness in yourself, which produces many positive effects. First, it helps you better understand and explore your thoughts so you can differentiate between your own emotions and those that you absorb from your abuser. Second, it helps you calm down your stressed nerves and respond to situations by thinking things through instead of impulsively reacting to them. This ensures you do not do anything yourself to trigger your abuser's volatile episodes, but you also seek appropriate ways to help him/her out and also escape the abuse inflicted upon you. Third, it helps you become more accepting of yourself and instead of bashing, belittling and disparaging yourself for keeping up with the codependent relationship for all this time, you forgive yourself, love yourself and move towards recovery and improvement. Moreover, it makes you more conscious towards your own needs encouraging you to engage more in self-care and self-love. To enjoy all these benefits, here is how you can practice mindfulness based meditation. While there are several ways to do it, this book will teach you a simple technique that works well for beginners: mindfulness based breathing meditation.

- Sit in a quiet, peaceful spot comfortably in any pose you like. You can sit on your yoga mat, a cushion, a chair, a couch or even lie down if sitting for 2 minutes is somehow uncomfortable.

- Set the timer for 2 minutes and close your eyes.

- Think of any happy memory that always makes you smile. It could be the first time you became a parent or your graduation day 6 years back or the time you went on a vacation to Maldives with friends.

- Reminisce the memory for a few moments and when it calms you down, slowly bring your attention, one bit at a time on your breath.

- Keep breathing in your natural manner even if it is rapid, but just inhale through your nose and exhale via your mouth.

- Your breath is going to be the object of your focus for 2 whole minutes so throughout this time, your goal is to watch your breath as you inhale and exhale.

- When you inhale, observe how it moves in your body and produces movements like the rising of your abdomen. Do the same when you exhale and this time, pay attention to the falling of your abdomen.

- Keep observing your breath and the many sensations it initiates in your body and you will find yourself becoming calmer with each breath you take.

- At some point, you may feel your attention breaking away to some other thought. It is okay if this happens because you are still adjusting to the idea of focusing on one thing at a time. Many of us do not have that ability and have the habit of thinking on multiple things simultaneously, which is why we do not have clarity on things. When you wander off in thought, very calmly, realign your attention back on your breath and start watching it again. If it helps, count your breath and tell yourself you will think about other tasks once these 2 minutes are over. Do this a few times and you will be okay.

- When your timer beeps, very gently, open your eyes and allow yourself a few moments to return to the real world. You are likely to feel quite fresh and relaxed than before. Bask in this beautiful feeling.

You need to practice this exercise twice daily for 2 to 5 minutes. In a couple of weeks after consistent practice, your focus will improve. Now is the time to focus on your thoughts by taking one thought or emotion at a time and meditating on it. You will be surprised at the insight it gives you. You will also become more aware of why you have been keeping up with this relationship for a long time, and will gain motivation from within to break this malicious cycle. Try to write down your feelings when you meditate on them to remember them and get more clarity on them. Also, this helps you communicate better with your abuser.

- ✓ Ask trusted friends how they view your communication and where they think you should

49

improve. An honest friend will readily tell you whether they normally believe you when you talk or whether they feel you are not communicating your true thoughts.

✓ Write down your thoughts, what you plan to do in the order of priority then track them down to progress. This exercise forces you to be truly honest with your thoughts and yourself. If you haven't achieved a plan you haven't and vice versa; no two ways about it.

✓ When you are better aware of how you feel about being in that relationship, find an appropriate time to talk to your abuser about them. It should be a time when he/ she is in a good mood, is speaking nicely to you and feels sane enough to listen to you. Casually go up to him/ her, and ask him/ her to sit down and then politely start talking about your feelings. Don't give them a heads up because sometimes when your abuser has a hunch about what you are going to talk about, he/ she is likely to go outside or throw a tantrum at the exact same time just to distract you from your motive and lure you into the codependency trap. It is quite likely he/ she is aware of his/ her dependency on your care and does not wish for the spiteful cycle to ever end because it is spiteful for you, but important and nurturing for them. If you inform him/ her beforehand that you wish to talk about something important with him/ her, he/ she is likely to avoid the talk. So it is best to look for a nice time to bring up the subject and take the plunge. Talk to him/ her in depth about your feelings, how being with him/ her suffocates you/ how all of this is affecting both of you negatively and how you wish to share a real, healthy and happy bond with him/ her. Also, let him/ her know that you are now strong enough to fight for your rights and will not take any nonsense from him/ her. If he/ she listens to you patiently and ends up accepting his/ her mistake while promising to behave better and work together on the relationship with you, it is okay to give it another chance. If, however, he/ she interrupts you in the middle, completely refuses to accept his/ her mistake and gaslights you again, it is clear he/ she only knows to control you and there is absolutely no point in wasting your time with him/ her. It is best to stay quiet at that time and work on your plan of leaving your abuser soon enough.

When you communicate your thoughts, others will also have to communicate their honest thoughts and feelings to you. Ideally, that forms the perfect relationship, one that is governed by honesty in self-expression. A firm self-identity and respect for others forms the basis for mutual respect and a healthy love relationship.

6: Identify and grow in a mutual relationship

Instead of a nurturing a dependent relationship, seek relationships with people who understand mutuality instead of dependency in a relationship. In a mutual relationship, each partner opens up to each other about their true feelings and emotions making it a relationship based on truth and openness instead of denial and sufferings.

You can learn to identify people who are independent in their thoughts after you have learnt to self-communicate effectively; essentially, when you detach fully from the bondage of codependency. Check out for the following characteristics in independent thinkers who understand mutual relationship.

✓ Allows you to speak your mind

✓ Takes turn to speak what they think

✓ You can easily draw a concrete answer or conclusion together owing to independent contribution of ideas

✓ You can learn something new from that person and you can prove its authenticity

7: Express your true thoughts and say 'no' where you truly feel is a no

Since you don't know how to say no, you know no boundaries. This puts you on a path that you cannot control yourself on. Learning to listen to your inner self will help you to set clear boundaries based on your values. Your partner will respect you for that.

In other words, do not feel coerced to serve anyone out of compulsion. Serve from the heart rather than from unwarranted fears of rejection or simply pleasing others.

Consider the repercussions and the benefits and act from a sober angle of reasoning. Before learning how to say a 'no' to your abuser, you first need to learn to set and establish healthy boundaries in a relationship.

✓ Spend some time reflecting on your core values, principles and beliefs and write them down. For example, if honesty is important to you in every aspect of your life, your core value could be to be honest in every relationship you engage in your life.

✓ Write down all your core values that you become aware of. With time, we change so it is okay if your core values change with time or you build new ones, but for now, write down all those that you believe in or all those that you would like to nurture. For instance, right now you may not have the habit of fighting for your rights, but you do wish to turn into someone who is aware of his/ her rights and stands up for them. So if you wish to become that person, write down that core value so you can work on it.

✓ Also, think of how you wish to be treated in different relationships and how you wish for the other person to behave with you. Take one relationship at a time and explore it in detail before moving to another one. Start off with the type of relationship you share with your abuser, and how you would like it to be different than what it is currently. List down all the things you wish for and want in that relationship keeping in mind the basic needs of the other person as well. If you do not wish to be yelled at, understand that maybe the need of the other person too.

✓ Once you have written out the majority of your core values and the things you would like to work on and build in a relationship, set boundaries based on it. If sincerity is a core value, a healthy boundary in your intimate relationship with your spouse could be that both of you must be sincere to each other and never resort to infidelity.

✓ Once the boundaries have been figured out, you need to go through them a few times to ensure you haven't missed out on anything important.

✓ Next, communicate those with the different people you share relationships with beginning with your abuser.

You then need to work on building the habit of saying no when needed because now you know what you must not compromise on.

Tips on how to say 'no':

✓ Understand that it is your right to say 'no' to your abuser when the need arises. Yes, you may not please partner by saying no, but you are not obliged to pay heed to every direction he/she throws your way. You are a free individual after all and are entitled to live your life on your terms. Caring and compromising occasionally is one thing, but allowing someone else to completely take over you and belittle you is completely unacceptable. So when you feel you must not give in to a certain whim or wish of your abuser, be firm, go ahead and say a 'NO.'

✓ Don't succumb to guilt of saying no. Initially, when you refuse to do something your abuser asks of you, you will feel guilty because you do not have the habit of behaving like that. You will feel bad for rejecting his wish even though a part of you wants to quickly jump up and agree to whatever he/ she wants. At this time, you need to act very rationally and think clearly. You have been taught how to breathe mindfully and stay in the moment. Practice mindfulness breathing meditation at that point by excusing yourself from the situation, or by staying there and taking a moment to get clarity on things. If you are sure you must say no to your abuser, do not allow guilt to wash you over. Remind yourself of your core values and how you are doing yourself a favor by sticking to them and not succumbing to the pressure created by your abuser. Think of how this one 'no' will pave way for many other 'No's' that you will utter because you do not wish to be treated like a doormat and avail your right of being a free individual. When you think of it this way, you feel less remorseful about declining a favor to your abuser. You then need to ensure to stick to this stance every time your abuser asks you to do something that is completely unacceptable to you. After a couple of attempts, you will get the hang of saying 'no' when something does not feel right and will feel quite confident about yourself. Also, your self-esteem will start improving because now you no longer view yourself as somebody's trash can as you have seen yourself stand up for yourself. Your abuser too, if he/she wishes to improve genuinely will become okay with you not agreeing to everything he/she says and will learn to accept your wishes too.

✓ Appreciate the offer, but state the reason for your denial clearly. Be keen also to state that you are keen to support in another way possible with you.

8: Don't fear to question

Don't languish with unanswered questions in your mind about your partner for the fear of rejection. Learn everything that is there to be learnt about your partner for openness and you'll be able to handle them well from a point of clear mutual understanding.

Some important things you may be interested in learning about your partner before you start a relationship include:

-Join a support group

Several support groups like Codependent Anonymous International, CoDA <u>coda.org,</u> Daily Strength <u>dailystrength.org</u> and many more online. Such give you insights on how best to recover. You also get to learn about others who are going through the same as you and give each other strength and ideas to overcome. But in case things don't really work out for you from support groups; you can back it up with a more one-on-one professional help.

-Seek professional help

As it is, resolving a deep-seated relationship problem that originated in childhood can be hard. But professionals have been trained on it and can persevere until you overcome.

But what does the help entail?

*Psychotherapy treatment for codependency

Therapists mostly help in administering a stricter approach to recovery. Most of the times, you don't realize the simple things you are doing that constitute to a codependent relationship.

A trained therapist will train you to identify the specific codependent tendencies so that it will be easier to drop them. Next, he/she will train you on the path to compassion and quickest route to recovery based on the findings of the specific codependent tendencies in you.

Next, we will be discussing how to caring for yourself to build your self-esteem.

Chapter 4: How To Start Caring For Yourself, Boosting Self Esteem

Once you are on the road to recovery from the harrowing relationship, you may feel you have been wasted or need some rebuilding. The first step to caring for oneself and build a solid life away from what you are used to is to:

1. **Completely reject to serving as the caregiver for other people's problems**

Unless it is life threatening or any other logical need for help, you need to refrain from your old helping tendencies. Don't let others use you with so many mundane requests.

Learn to give your partner space to try to deal with their problems and see the magic this works. People will respect you for that and with time, you will nurture your relationship into mutuality where each partner contributes.

You now know how to set healthy boundaries in relationships so put that information to use and build new bonds while setting meaningful and healthy boundaries in them so you allow nobody to become your boss and can focus on establishing a happy, meaningful relationship with them. After you have built healthy boundaries in a relationship and have the other person come up to you for a need or a favor that you find objectionable, be strong and refuse it.

Also, ensure not to take up on your caregiver role ever again in any other relationship even when you experience a strong urge to do so. Take deep breaths in that time by inhaling to a count of 5, holding the breath to another count of 5 and then exhaling to a final count of 5. Do that for 10 to 20 times and you will feel relaxed, more focused and mindful which will help you make a rational decision. Also, remind yourself of how being an absolute caregiver turned out for you in your last abusive relationship and how you do not wish to relive that experience again.

Hence, it is best to look after yourself first and not jump into being someone else's guardian and ruin your life once again.

2. Find healthy hobbies

Remember that you have had a long time of self-denial and have not focused on your own needs for quite a long time. Finding something you enjoy to do is very important to start connecting with your emotions and self-fulfillment.

If you find it difficult identifying the activity you like, sit down and try brainstorming on what you value. Any game, is it fishing, is it hiking, going on bike tour, jogging, stone collecting etc. what it that intrigues you? List them down and you will soon discover where your interests lie. Go on with the activity and discover the fulfillment in it.

You need to build habits of those activities by turning them into rituals. Try one activity at a time and see how it makes you feel. If you decide to go on a hike, observe your feelings throughout the experience and if it is a liberating, gratifying, thrilling and enjoyable experience, and one that you would like to experience again, turn it into a weekly or bi-monthly experience. Similarly, if painting relaxes you, you could do it every weekend.

Your goal should be to do something calming, exciting, enjoyable and meaningful every single day even if it is just reading a book for 15 minutes. There needs to be a certain part of the day that you devote only to yourself and nothing else so you actually feel good about yourself from within, and feel that your life really is about you; otherwise, you will just think of yourself as a robot who jumps from one chore to another mechanically.

3. Do not procrastinate

Remember that your stay in a codependent relationship was a very busy and structured one. It's so ingrained in you, you were so used to it and slightest chances of boredom or letting your guards off can find you slipping back to it. Ensure that you stop catering to others people's problems now. Start an activity that you enjoy now.

Nonetheless, approach the change gradually, one step at a time. The first day can be spent on just trying to figure out your hobby, second day could be about researching a bit about it. Third day, find the best way to start and then start gradually. The point is keep your thoughts busy with something that relates to you.

Remember, like any other addiction, abrupt change from what you were used to can frustrate your efforts of stopping. The point is to make constant gradual steps, everyday towards a complete change.

4. Take care of your health

It is not only your emotional needs that you have ignored all this time while being in a codependent relationship. You also completely overlooked your physical health and wellbeing, and paid no attention to your eating habits, nutrition, sleep routine and fitness needs. It is likely you used to stay up late for hours, toss and turn in bed because you weren't happy, did not eat properly, ate too much or too little, did not eat healthy foods, lived a very sedentary lifestyle or were too active that you worked out your body way too much and only harmed it in the end.

You now need to improve on these practices and start taking better care of yourself. Start off by doing the following:

✓ Take an in depth of account of your eating habits and routine. Do you skip your breakfast? Do you eat whatever you can find in the fridge or consume processed and packaged foods regularly because you are always too tired to prepare a home cooked meal yourself? Does your diet not contain any healthy, fresh and whole foods? Do you eat too much at a single time? Do you often eat even when you don't feel like eating just to shove food on top of your feelings to feel less stressed? If you do all of that, you are not taking care of yourself and need to do better.

✓ Slowly incorporate more fresh fruits, veggies, lean meat cuts, whole wheat grains and foods, dairy products, nuts and seeds in your diet and replace all the processed and packaged foods rich in trans-fats, genetically modified organisms (GMOs), artificial flavors and ingredients and processed sugar with those foods. Make sure to have at least one healthy and home cooked meal a day.

✓ Never skip your breakfast and make sure to make it the healthiest meal of your day. Eat a piece or two of fruit with an egg, two slices of bread and a bowl of cereal. You can have tea or coffee alongside, and ensure to eat with a gap of maximum 90 minutes after you wake up.

✓ Your lunch needs to be not too heavy and your dinner needs to be light. Make sure to have a healthy snack in between your main meals and have 5 to 6 small portioned meals throughout the day instead of having really big 2 or 3 meals.

✓ Drink at least 2.5 liters of clean, drinking water daily to stay hydrated and fresh. Also, it keeps you thinking actively and make good decisions.

✓ Stay active throughout the day by doing your chores yourself and walking, taking the stairs and jogging lightly whenever possible.

✓ Work out for 15 to 60 minutes during the day by doing anything exciting and rigorous that you enjoy. You can do Pilates, yoga, kickboxing, swim, play a sport, dance or just brisk walk.

✓ Do not work out when your tummy is too full or right before your sleep time as it can lead to tummy aches and disrupt your sleep cycle, respectively.

✓ Set a sleep and waking time, and ensure to go to bed at that very time every night. You need to wake up at the wake time too even if you could not sleep properly the entire night. Do this for a few days and soon, your body and mind will adjust to this new cycle.

✓ Keep your phone and other screens away an hour before your bed time and do something soothing instead to initiate sleep easily. Blue rays emitted by the screens disrupt your circadian cycle making it difficult for you to initiate and maintain sleep at night.

✓ Also, ensure that your bed and pillows are soft enough to relax you and do not trigger any body pain so you sleep comfortably on them.

✓ Dim the lights in the room and switch off any noisy appliances around to sleep peacefully through the night.

✓ Work out 3 to 4 hours before your sleep time to work out your muscles. When your body is tired, you go to bed on time easily.

✓ During mid-day, take a nap of 10 to 60 minutes to rejuvenate your body and energize it for the next round of chores.

Work on these tips and soon, you will feel much better about yourself. When you provide your body and mind with enough care and rest, the right nutrition and activity, you feel strong and fit from within, which also makes it easier for you think rationally.

If you work on all the strategies discussed in this chapter, you will slowly find yourself becoming stronger, confident and powerful with time ready to face the world and will recover from the trauma you underwent as well.

Next, our focus will be on when to consider separation.

Stop Codependency

Chapter 5: Considering Separation to Detangle You From Codependence

One of the likely options available at your disposal to end the suffering experienced in a codependent relationship is to break it off. You have done all that is possible to change your partner, but nothing is forthcoming, and things have escalated even to life threatening levels and now you don't have an option, but to separate with your partner.

Like many other painful consequential relationships breakups, this is also never an easy option neither is it legally abiding in some cases. The impact of separation is also sometimes unbearable.

For example, your partner out of his behaviors seems to be punishing you without any reason. He has become an unruly alcoholic and you feel this is taking a toll on your family. Maybe he has turned a narcissist, treating you with disrespect, disregard and manipulates you despite your efforts to try and support him. The world can clearly see there is a big problem and you are so guilty that it is the problem in your house and you are the sober one and you are not helping. As a viable option, you seek help for your partner but still nothing is changing. The children are suffering and helpless.

It looks as if (or so you think) they are doing so because you aren't intervening to help. He or she even starts becoming abusive. Very well knowing the repercussions of initiating a codependent relationship to become an enabler, you can't help it to help to start caring for your partner unfortunately initiating a codependency cycle. It is the only option left.

After a long struggle with an abusive partner, he or she suddenly vanishes without warning. After searching and enduring unexplained bad treatment from them, you almost give up on the relationship. But then the lost partner reappears from nowhere probably looking even more beaten and vengeful. At some point, they even threaten suicide or murder.

Once again, you wonder what wrong you ever committed to deserve this treatment. Again, you reconsider the codependent role of taking care of them at least to weaken their nerve of anger and fury.

However, it is never worth sliding back to a codependence relationship. It's as unnerving as the bad treatment or even worse. You can't stand the pain and suffering and you close to breaking point. At the breaking point, you consider breakup from the relationship.

Resort to Your Break-Up Plan

Remember, the plan you were asked to craft with your supportive buddy to escape the abusive relationship? It is time to take that out and implement it for real. One fine day when he/she is way, leave the place and switch off your current number. Switch to the new number you have hidden with your friend. If you are scared of your abuser approaching you, inform the police and consult your lawyer right away.

In case you are afraid of him/ her finding out your safe haven, do not crash at your friend's place and resort to a shelter home he/ she is unaware of for a few days. You should also consider getting a restraining order against him/ her, especially if you are sure he/ she will opt for volatile means to deal with you.

When you do break it up with your abuser, remember to toss out all the things you have of him/ her and those that remind you of your time spent with that person. There is no point in carrying any physical baggage along with the emotional one that may weigh you down emotionally so just let go if to allow peace to flow inside you.

Dealing With Codependence In Your Long-Term Relationship Where You Feel You Cannot Break Up

One of the most challenging aspects of a codependency relationship is when you do not have an option, but to stay in an abusive relationship. For example, you are bound by marriage vows and you have children.

You can see the marriage is clearly coming to an end but you simply can't initiate the breakup. Or for instance, if you have a child who is a drug addict and you cannot bring yourself to the point to leave him/ her.

In such cases, you can try to once again improve the other person by improving yourself. If you become firmer and stricter with them, it is likely they will improve.

However, if that does not help, there is nothing wrong or sinful about leaving that abusive person even if he/ she is your spouse. You can get the custody of your kids and leave him/ her because children raised in an abusive marriage end up having problems themselves. As for a drug addict kid or partner, you can get them admitted in a rehabilitation center and make sure they complete their program.

Conclusion

We have come to the end of the book. Congratulations for reading until the end. It shows you have real commitment to transform your life positively.

As it is evident, codependency is a very serious problem that needs eradication. Separation is never the best option due to the negative impact likely worse than enduring the relationship. Recovery approach is the answer. You also may be keen to realize that its onset in a relationship is never obvious. It's so gradual and before you know, the cycle is so mature, in its third turn. Always watch out for the slightest indication of it in a relationship and quickly employ a no more attack to counter the malady.

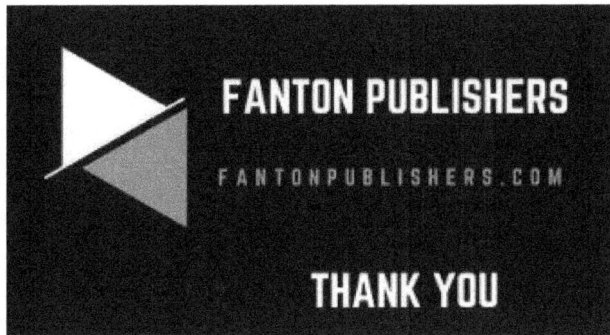

FANTON PUBLISHERS

FANTONPUBLISHERS.COM

THANK YOU

Do You Like My Book & Approach To Publishing?

If you like my writing and style and would love the ease of learning literally everything you can get your hands on from Fantonpublishers.com, I'd really need you to do me either of the following favors.

1: First, I'd Love It If You Leave a Review of This Book on Amazon.

2: Check Out My Emotional Mastery Books

<u>Emotional Intelligence: The Mindfulness Guide To Mastering Your Emotions, Getting Ahead And Improving Your Life</u>

<u>Stress: The Psychology of Managing Pressure: Practical Strategies to turn Pressure into Positive Energy (5 Key Stress Techniques for Stress, Anxiety, and Depression Relief)</u>

<u>Failure Is Not The END: It Is An Emotional Gym: Complete Workout Plan On How To Build Your Emotional Muscle And Burning Down Anxiety To Become Emotionally Stronger, More Confident and Less Reactive</u>

<u>Subconscious Mind: Tame, Reprogram & Control Your Subconscious Mind To Transform Your Life</u>

[Body Language: Master Body Language: A Practical Guide to Understanding Nonverbal Communication and Improving Your Relationships](#)

[Shame and Guilt: Overcoming Shame and Guilt: Step By Step Guide On How to Overcome Shame and Guilt for Good](#)

[Anger Management: A Simple Guide on How to Deal with Anger](#)

Get updates when we publish any book that will help you master your emotions: http://bit.ly/2fantonpubpersonaldevl

To get a list of all my other books, visit my author profile or let me send you the list by requesting them below: http://bit.ly/2fantonpubnewbooks

3: Grab Some Freebies On Your Way Out; Giving Is Receiving, Right?

I gave you a complimentary book at the start of the book. If you are still interested, grab it here.

[5 Pillar Life Transformation Checklist](#): http://bit.ly/2fantonfreebie